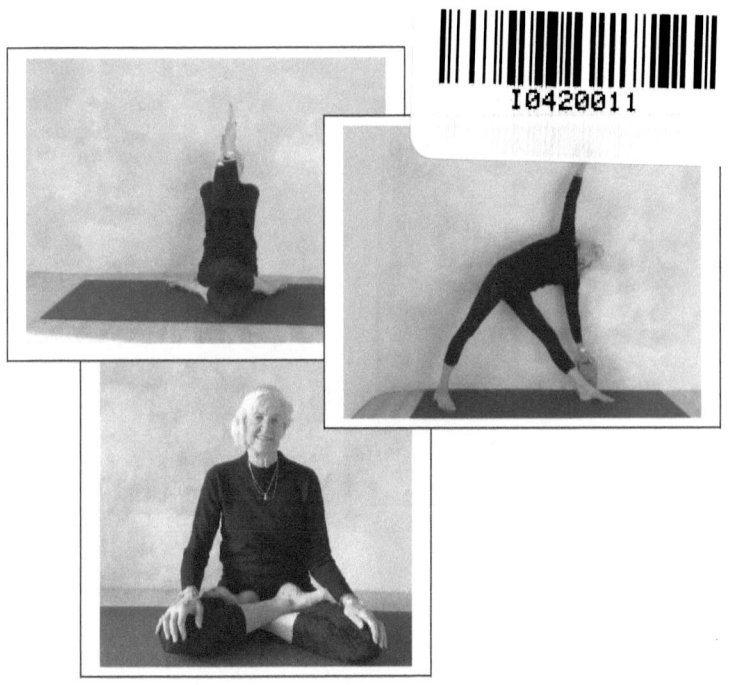

The Principles

of Yoga

for Beginners

by Felicity Green

This book is dedicated to

the loving memory of

B.K.S. Iyengar

Yoga aims for complete awareness in everything you do.

B.K.S. Iyengar

Introduction

Yoga is an ancient system for the development of our human nature. The highest pinnacle of our life is to be totally aware and alive, and in the present. Yoga was postulated by Patanjali, the Indian Sage who compiled the Yoga Sutras.

Although Patanjali lived in India 7,000 years ago, the human condition is still the same; we are all seeking happiness, love and contentment.

His Sutras, of which there are 4 books, are a timeless guide to develop your character and to help you become a deeply authentic and vibrant person.

Having an understanding of the Principles of Yoga, this 7,000 year old study of linking body, mind, and soul, will greatly enhance your practice. Interweaving an understanding of the Principles of Yoga with the Asana—yoga positions—will greatly increase the rewards of your effort.

I have simplified these principles so in your practice you can explore your body in relation to these principles. The goal of this book—as is the goal of Yoga—is for YOU to live a healthy, happy and content life.

Yoga is the harmony of the body, senses, mind, and intellect; that's why there is no difference between physical and mental yoga.

B.K.S. Iyengar

The Eight Limbs of Patanjali Yoga Sutras

Many Westerners think that Asana is the first step to a yoga practice. The truth is that in the Eight Limbs of Patanjali's Yoga Lineage the ethical ways of living are first. These principles are first learned in your body. Yamas, Niyamas and Asana create a broad foundation for later benefits of wisdom and peace and contentment.

- **Yamas**: relation to the world and others
- **Niyamas**: relation to yourself
- **Asana**: bodily postures
- **Pranayama**: breath control
- **Pratyahara**: controlled use of the senses
- **Dharana**: focus on a broad subject
- **Dhyana**: complete focus
- **Samadhi**: a loss of ego self

The first two, Yamas and Niyamas are yoga ethics. Asana, Pranayama and Pratyahara are the external practices. Dharana, Dhyana, and Samadhi are the internal practices.

"Learn to do your ABC's before you try to do your PhD." B.K.S. Iyengar

INSTRUCTIONS:

1. Read the questions with personal pronouns.
2. Answer each question with the personal pronoun from your physical, mental and emotion perspective.
3. Repeat this throughout the book and review every three months. This will help you notice how you are beginning to change.
4. Use the Notes section to observe your progress. Filling in your awareness with the date will give you a marker of your progress.

Yamas

The Yamas are how we interact with society and other people.

Consider these five principles in your relationships to yourself and others.

Ahimsa

1. **Ahimsa** / Non-violence

In thought, word and deed.
To be aware of not being loving,
even to yourself.

In your asana do you understand where the
boundary is between over stretching or not
challenging yourself enough to connect
mind to body?

Do you injure yourself
in Asana practice?

Do you have negative or critical thoughts
about yourself
during your practice?

When you are annoyed
are your words hurtful to others ?

What is your attitude toward other
forms of life?

Satya

NOTES: **DATE:**

2. Satya / Non lying

In thought word and deed.

The truth is so much easier. Otherwise you have to remember the untruth and who you told it to. Being honest with yourself is the most important way to become authentic.

Satya is the lynch pin of ethics.

Are you honest about your body, where it is flexible and where weak?

Is this the result of the use of your body in the past?

Do you need to change old habits; physically, mentally, emotionally?

Brahmacharya

NOTES: **DATE:**

3. **Brahmacharya** / Moderation

Brahma is the Creator;
Acharya is to walk with,
to live ethically.

So practice with awareness
And with a grateful
and devotional attitude.

Do you take care of your body as a temple
for your spirit?

Are you moderate in the different aspects
of your life:
Eating, sleeping, exercising,
working and relaxation?

Are you moderate in your
use of energy:
physically, mentally,
emotionally?

Asteya

NOTES: **DATE:**

4. **Asteya** / Non-Stealing

Not taking what
belongs to others.

There are many ways to steal
other than materially:

Do you take credit for ideas
that are not your own?

Are the stronger areas of your body stealing
from the weak ones?

Do you steal somebody's
self-esteem with unkind words?

The joy of living can be stolen
by our negative attitudes,
and a fear of accepting challenges.

Aparigraha

NOTES: **DATE:**

5. Aparigraha / Non-Coveting

Respect for what belongs to others.

"Have what you need and

use what you have. "

-B.K.S Iyengar

Accepting your present circumstances does
not mean you become complacent--
contentment is in the moment.

Are you being introspective
in your practice?

Are you in touch with feelings in
your own body and not comparing
yourself to others?

Do you find contentment and gratitude
for the body you have?

In Yoga the belief is that humans have 5 sheaths—
Kosas—or layers that make up the whole human being.

These sheaths represent the 5 elements of nature:

Earth, Water, Fire and Ether

B.K.S. Iyengar

1) The Anatomical Body—Anamayakosa--
   Your muscles and bones
2) The Energy Body— Pranamayakosa
   All the systems in your body; like your
   respiration, circulation, etc.
3) The Mental/Emotional Body—
   Manomayakosa. What you think and feel
4) The Wisdom Body—Vijnanamayakosa
   The enhanced awareness that these practices
   bring.
5) The Spiritual Body—Anadamayakosa
   That aspect that is peaceful and content.

As you work with (1) your muscles and bones, you
cannot but affect (2) your breathing and circulation and
all your organs. Then as you do your Asana—yoga
positions—and focus your mind, you affect (3) your
mental/emotional body, and most often the way you
experience life emotionally will change. And, this
affects your spiritual body—Anamayakosa.

When you apply the Yamas and Niyamas to all three of
your external aspects you begin to develop wisdom.

Niyamas

**The Niyamas are how
we relate to ourselves.**

Consider these five principles and find
out where and when you are not
abiding to them, and where you would
choose to live differently.

Saucha

NOTES: **DATE:**

1. **Saucha** / Cleanliness

Keeping, clean physically, not just exteriorly but internally by eating healthy, fresh food and drinking fresh water.

Live in an uncluttered space.

Be careful not to pollute yourself with negative influences, but keep good company and have enough sleep.

Do you have clarity and concentration in your asana practice?

Do you walk your talk in your relationships with others?

Do you use your imagination to create positive thoughts, as opposed to negative ones?

On reflection on your actions, are you accountable and do you behave responsibly?

Santosa

2. **Santosa** / Contentment

To be happy and grateful to be alive with what is now in the present.

Accept that, but know that everything changes. You may be feeling content, and then something happens to change the circumstances and you are suddenly no longer content.

Life is pain and pleasure; suffering is the mental continuation of pain.

Contentment is the cultivation of well-being in each moment.

When you are well balanced you feel free in your asana as well as in your life.

What makes you feel content?

What is the difference between complacency and contentment?

Tapas

3. **Tapas** / Effort

Tapas relate to you having passion, fiery discipline and commitment to your ideals and direction in life.

"The tapas of asana develops will"

B.K.S. Iyengar

Asana is how you get rid of some the knots and tangles in your body, which are unresolved emotional or physical difficulties often coming from your previous experiences.

Asana is your main practice of tapas at this time.

This may involve letting go of security and having the courage to face your fears and create change.

What Asanas do you avoid or are you afraid of? Practice them.

What Asanas have an emotional content? Practice them.

Svadhyaya

4. Svadhyaya / Self-study

Svadhyaya is an examination of yourself through introspective practices.

"An unexamined life is a life not worth living."

Voltaire

Giving yourself enough time to see yourself in relation to these ten mirrors of the Yamas and Niyamas.

Look at yourself honestly. Write about your thoughts and speech to become more aware of areas where you could change your attitude.

Use writing periodically to investigate your Asanas?

What did you learn this time? Note it.

What words or thoughts make you not like yourself?

Ishvara Pranidhana

NOTES: **DATE:**

5. Ishvara Pranidhana / Devotion

The name of this Higher power doesn't matter, different groups have varied names but they all mean that we have an acknowledgment of this Higher Power.

Do you have belief in a higher power that supports you positively as you tread the road of your life?

Do you practice your asana with joyful awareness?

Are you a person who believes you are in total control of your life?

Do you realize that your ego is not who you are?

Do you have a devotional practice?

Think Light!

Try to impart a feeling of lightness to the body. Think light. This can be achieved by mentally extending yourself outwards from the center of our body, i.e. think tall. Think not just of raising your arms but of extending them outwards and when you are holding them still, think again of reaching still further away from your body.

Do not think of yourself as a small compressed suffering thing. Think of yourself as graceful and expanding – no matter how unlikely it may seem at the time.

B.K.S. Iyengar

Blessings

Your personal practice should be regular, at least 5 days a week. Start slowly, 15 minutes a day is worth much more than an hour and a half twice a week. Try to practice at the same time and the same place as much as possible.

Put your practice at the top of your list; don't try to fit it into the cracks of your life. Sometimes the body is willing but the mind is not.

"Don't worry, just practice."

B.K.S. Iyengar

When you have practiced faithfully and consistently for about 3 years it is time to tackle Pranayama. This is the interface between your physical body and your mind and emotions. B.K.S.Iyengar called this the Hub of Yoga.

This is a self-adjusting system: there is no sin in Yoga. You choose how to live your life.

If we were all able to live in accordance with the Yamas and Niyamas, this would be a perfect world, as all our relationships with ourselves and others would be based on love and consideration.

Blessings on your journey,
Felicity Green
Advanced Iyengar Teacher
Revised by Liz Lafferty 2017